D1553875

Bone Health Made Easy

Ultrasound Bone Density Testing:
Why Most People Should Have It Done *Now*,
And Have It Done More Often Than Ever!

Kenneth C. Howayeck, D.P.M.
Osteoporosis Educator

First Edition

ISBN: 978-0-615-48639-0

Editor: Dalya F. Massachi/Writing for Community Success
Book design: Erin McReynolds

Printed in the United States of America

About the Author

Dr. Kenneth C. Howayeck currently resides in Alameda, California,
where he works as an Osteoporosis
Public Educator and Osteoporosis
Education Specialist. He has au-
thored two other books, *My Foot Is
Killing Me!* and *Effective Actions*. In
2001, he hosted "Foot Notes," a radio
talk show in Honolulu, Hawaii.

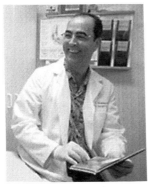

During his distinguished 22-
year career in Hawaii, Dr. Howayeck
specialized in podiatry and podiatric surgery. He also served
as Assistant Clinical Professor of Surgery at the University
of Hawaii School of Medicine, and oversaw surgery in the
Surgical Fellowship program that he founded at HealthSouth
Surgical Center. In addition, he served as President of the
Hawaii Podiatric Medical Association from 1996-1997.

While in private practice, Dr. Howayeck diagnosed and
treated osteoporosis-related fragility stress fractures of the
foot, and interpreted thousands of ultrasound bone density
tests. Sadly, in June 2010, he lost his own mother six weeks
after an osteoporosis-related hip fracture. These experiences
prompted him to leverage his professional background to
promote public education around the horrible and widely
understated issues surrounding osteoporosis.

In May of 2010, Dr. Howayeck founded Five Star Testing
Service, which brings accessible ultrasound bone density
screening to various employers and community wellness
events (see Appendix D, page 45 for more information). He
also serves as a private anti-aging consultant and personal
medical and podiatry coach. In addition, he is a Certified
Speaker for the Foundation for Osteoporosis Research & Education and the San Francisco Bay Area chapter of American
Bone Health.

In Dedication

I dedicate this book to my lovely wife, Margaret: You do so much for me. Always have. Without you, none of this could happen. You not only help me, but you also inspire me. You believe so much in me. I love you. Through many tough times, and with many dreams, you have always loved the real me. You truly want me to enjoy life, to be happy, and to always be with you.

And to my daughters, Katrina and Nila: I truly wish the same for you. I think of you every day. You should dream, and I dream for you. I also dream of you, and dream of all of us being together. I love you.

ACKNOWLEDGMENTS

So many people have done so much for me with absolutely no expectations attached, and at times with little given in return for their kindness.

I must first thank my mother, who was once Ann Louise Mendes, who always believed in me, and who loved me very, very much. She often said to me to never sell myself short. She was always there for me when a softer and more reasonable buffer was needed. I love her. I miss her. I feel her with me.

Several others have been instrumental in my learning and thinking processes, many of which have led to this book. I cannot possibly mention them all.

I also want to thank Telesha Klee. She did so much for me, for so long, by making sure I was equipped to do so many bone density screenings—simply out of her own kindness and generosity. And I know that she certainly did not have to.

In addition, I want to thank my editor, Dalya Massachi, for all her assistance and understanding in the production of this book. It was no small undertaking, and she did a great job.

"Do what you love. Know your own bone; gnaw at it, bury it, unearth it, and gnaw it still."
— *Henry David Thoreau*

Table of Contents

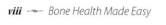

"To be the lone voice in a crowd does not make one wrong."
— Mahatma Gandhi

Top Nine Osteoporosis Jaw-Droppers

#9: At six months following a hip fracture—all hip fractures, mind you--- only about 15% of people are able to walk across a room unaided. This fact suggests that a hip fracture is no normal fracture to get! And yet, the hip is often the area that fractures when osteoporosis exists.[1]

#8: One in five of those who could walk before their hip fracture require long-term care afterward.[2]

#7: Half of all people suffering from a hip fracture from osteoporosis will never walk again.[3]

#6: Half of all women and up to one quarter of men over 50 will experience an osteoporosis-related stress fracture in their lifetime.[4]

#5: Four times as many men and nearly three times as many women have osteoporosis than report having the disease.[5]

---

1 National Osteoporosis Foundation: http://nof.org/node/40
2 Ibid
3 Ibid
4 Ibid
5 Office of the Surgeon General: ww.surgeongeneral.gov/library/bonehealth/factsheet1.html

#4: Hip fractures deriving from osteoporosis in women out-number deaths from breast, uterine, and ovarian cancers combined. In men, the incidences of hip fractures from osteoporosis outnumber deaths from prostate cancer, as well.[6]

#3: 24% of people over 50 who experience a hip fracture are dead within 12 months.[7]

#2: By 2050, the worldwide incidence of hip fracture is projected to increase by 310% in men, and 240% in women. (We are talking about our kids here!)[8]

#1: A 2005 study by researchers with Cornell University found that bone density screenings were associated with 36% fewer hip fractures over a six-year period, when compared with usual medical care.[9]

(Note: All source websites contained the cited statistics in Dec. 2010.)

---

6 National Osteoporosis Foundation: http://nof.org/node/40
7 Ibid
8 International Osteoporosis Foundation: http://www.iofbonehealth.org/facts-and-statistics.html
9 New York-Presbyterian Hospital/Weill Cornell Medical Center: http://bit.ly/gptfsc

1

Important Initial Notes

IMPORTANT INITIAL NOTES

Of course, you should see your doctor—about many things. And you should ask your doctor about how bone density (bone strength) loss might relate to you. You both should discuss this issue early in the process (rather than later). But ultimately, you are the one most responsible for your health.

You may know that DXA ("Dual energy X-ray absorptiometry") is typically and legitimately accepted in the U.S. as the definitive method of measuring bone mineral density. It is an expensive, high-tech medical procedure that brings out the big guns to fully evaluate the bone density situation. To have a DXA scan done, you typically must see a doctor—your own doctor, if possible. And you must get her or his order to do the test.

However, we have a much less expensive, lower-tech option that should precede DXA and can identify many more people at serious risk of getting osteoporosis: ultrasound bone density testing (UBDT). Unfortunately, your doctor is not nearly as likely to direct you to also get frequent ultrasound monitoring of your bone strength.

DXA is often the first—and only—method used to screen for bone density issues. UBDT is often bypassed. In fact, the U.S. Food and Drug Administration only approved ultrasound bone density testing equipment for commercial use in 1998. Many countries in Europe, Asia, and Latin America had already been using UBDT for some time, and the technology continues to be much more prevalent there.

You need to know about UBDT

I believe that everyone deserves great health. And that includes those who are not fitting perfectly well into our medical delivery system. Because it can reach many more people than DXA can, I believe that UBDT better addresses the obvious reasons that many people do not recognize and treat their bone density deficiency: finances, fears, time or scheduling problems, and certain belief systems. I have heard them all in my 22 years of clinical practice! This situation is varied, quite prevalent, and underestimated and misunderstood.

Clearly, UBDT cannot do the extensive evaluation that DXA can. DXA can target the hip, spine, forearm, wrist, and, in some cases, the heel bone. It can also target, and monitor through serial comparison, specific regions within these bones. UBDT almost always targets only the heel (the most important of all bones to target during initial screening).

However, DXA is incapable from a practical standpoint of achieving all of what UBDT can do to reach the majority of people in a more realistic, appealing, and effective manner.

Take a closer look

Is it possible that in the U.S. we are simply trying to make human beings fit our existing osteoporosis detection system (which is almost exclusively based on DXA), rather than adapting our medical approach to fit the needs of the human being? I believe this is the case.

But can individuals, or the system itself, really afford that approach? On many levels—and across the board—this certainly invites concern. In the absence of a commonplace testing standard for bone density, many people in need of screening are clearly not being tested. And many people's lives are at stake here! (Be sure to read the "Top Nine Osteo-porosis Jaw-Droppers" on page 9.)

Much of what I suggest in this book—while backed either by evidence or by simple reasoning—is not necessarily supported by some major institutions currently promoting osteoporosis awareness. But I, and others as well, feel quite strongly about what you are about to read.

"Go gently to the very bone. Find there a truth that is nearer and useful. It is ancient, to be revered. Hidden, until now."
— *Unknown*

Ultrasound Bone Density Testing (UBDT): The Basics

I believe Ultrasound Bone Density Testing (UBDT) has been extremely underutilized—at a time when we need it the most. The technology has developed tremendously in the past several years, through enhanced accuracy, speed, and even the amount of information that it now provides via displays and printouts. Unfortunately, UBDT is still not widely well-understood or appreciated for its actual purpose and potential.

ASK DR. KEN

I have never heard the term "UBDT." What is it?

"Ultrasound Bone Density Testing," or "UBDT," is the term I use to describe the process of screening or monitoring bone density. Bone density is the amount of bone tissue in a certain volume of bone. It is often associated with bone strength. UBDT provides a measurement of bone mineral density to indicate resistance to bone fracture (the "T-Score").

Keep in mind that UBDT is not DXA ("Dual energy X-ray absorptiometry"), which is done by X-Ray and must be ordered by a doctor.

I use the term "UBDT" because I believe it is much more accessible and easy-to-understand (and say) than the other terms in use today by medical professionals. You probably have never heard of the technical terms: "Quantitative Ultra-Sonography" (QUS) or "Peripheral Ultrasound Densitometry." Now is the time for a major re-focus of outreach efforts to everyone who may have weak bones. And that begins with a name change.

ASK DR. KEN

Why is it important to screen or monitor bone density?

A very low bone density T-score is equated with a higher risk of ultimately suffering from a bone break (or "fracture"). A significant risk for fracture typically suggests a higher risk of experiencing a spine, wrist, pelvic, foot, or—most ominously—hip fracture. When a hip fracture occurs, dramatic and unwanted factors come into play. Compressive forces begin on various important organs, and your body systems basically go haywire. From that, an extremely detrimental and rapid "metabolic cascade" begins to advance, compromising your ability to be comfortable and independent. Hip fracture patients have great difficulty moving and find that their entire life soon changes. Results? Some very negative health risks come into play (see "Top Nine Osteoporosis Jaw-Droppers" on page 9).

You need to know your level of risk. Breaking a bone can have disastrous consequences for your health, especially if you are over the age of 50. And UBDT can determine that risk, in an appealing and practical way. This type of awareness will influence your behavior choices. And yes, you can do some things to improve your T-score (read on to see what you can do). Armed with a UBDT report, you and your doctor can decide on next steps about how to improve your bone health, and in turn decrease your risks both now and in the future—for yourself and your loved ones!

Ask Dr. Ken

What does it mean to "screen" for bone density loss?

To screen is to sift or sort. Think of a screen at your window, door, or in your kitchen. We first must lead something (like air or flour) right through the screen. By doing so, we end up holding certain things back, or separating them, so as to point them out—and appropriately so.

In this case, screening helps identify people at risk for an ominous fracture, so we can focus attention on their needs and properly protect them. They are likely candidates for bone density loss and need further evaluation. Screening is searching for disease before symptoms are present.

UBDT is meant for, and has always been meant for, screening. That is what it's good at!

To be sure, bone density screening does not yield a complete or definitive diagnosis—nor is it intended to. That is why a troublesome UBDT result (T-score) should lead to a more thorough DXA test. But many people would otherwise have no idea that they were even at risk until their UBDT result tells them so.

Ask Dr. Ken

What advantages over DXA does UBDT have as a first screen for bone density deficiency?

I like to us the acronym *SCREEN*:

Simplicity (It doesn't get any simpler!)

Candidacy that is enhanced (In other words, many more people can justifiably undergo it)

Repeat-ability in many ways, for various reasons, with no risk

Expense is lower, using ultrasound instead of larger, more
expensive DXA equipment

Expedited process—a great deal so (that is, it's fast!)

NO harm—plain and simple – even from over-utilizing
this method

ASK DR. KEN

How Safe is UBDT?

UBDT is very safe. In fact, it is even safer than DXA. And
DXA, with much less radiation than that of a standard X-Ray,
is already quite safe. Ultrasound involves no radiation—just
sound that is not picked up by the ears of humans or most
other mammals.

Here is a way of understanding just how safe ultrasound
is: When determining the gender of a fetus, what do we turn
to? Ultrasound. Where is it placed and then what is it aimed
at? A pregnant woman's belly and directly at a fetus. We certainly would not take chances in that circumstance!

It is no wonder that state regulatory agencies find no
reason to assign the need for an operator's license or creden-
tialing for the operation of ultrasound machines. The process
resembles someone using a camera to simply click away to
obtain a visual image of another person.

The only cautionary note is that UBDT should not be
used over metallic hardware, as doing so could both skew the
measured result and perhaps increase the temperature of the
hardware a bit.

ASK DR. KEN

How does UBDT work?

UBDT simply involves a small machine that uses ultrasound to quickly and comfortably measure bone mineral

density—and thus your risk for bone fracture. Place your bare foot into the machine (some units use your wrist, forearm, or toes, instead). Sit still. In two to three minutes the test is complete! A report showing the result, which can be copied and provided to your doctor, is available to you immediately.

My particular bias is toward the UBDT of the foot, as opposed to using the wrist, forearm, or the toes. But no matter what part of the body gets scanned, for valid monitoring and comparison purposes I highly recommend the consistency afforded by repeatedly scanning exactly the same area of the body, using the very same machine, and even having the same operator. While this may not always be easy to do, comparing apples to apples should be the goal.

Ask Dr. Ken

When should I have UBDT done?

If you have not had a DXA or UBDT done in the last six months, it is at least helpful and interesting—if not wise—to take the time to do it now. Certainly, take advantage of its availability if you are aware of UBDT being offered in your area at an upcoming time. If you have gone much longer than six months since your last bone density screening, it is time to actively seek out a convenient location where UBDT is being offered. Do it often. Have it done much more often than most others are recommending. (Chapter 4 goes into this issue in greater detail).

Ask Dr. Ken

Can I still have a DXA down the line?

Of course you can—and should! A UBDT measurement, in the interim, will not get in the way. In fact, it will provide you and your doctor with more comprehensive information about your bone health than DXA's alone. And if you have never had a DXA, but your UBDT result indicates a potential bone density deficiency, you should definitely get a DXA.

The rest of this book will guide you through all you need to know about making UBDT work for you.

ASK DR. KEN:
Why Should Most People Consider
Frequent UBDT?

[Before I list my top 13 practical reasons, let me ask *you*: How many reasons do you need to consider doing something wise for yourself? Especially if it is something interesting, quick, and inexpensive?]

1. Why not?   (Yes, why not? "Why not" is a reason.) We are talking about you, right? You will probably find it helpful to be able to keep that last T-score—a pretty simple number in fact—in your head, right? Suppose you want to beat it? Suppose someone asks you what your T-score is? Don't worry about "over-using" UBDT; the potential positive effects of doing that far outweigh any added expenditure of money, time, effort, and perhaps confusion from information overload. Yet, all of those seem quite minimal when you are trying to assess and monitor your bone density. So...with no good reason to avoid doing UBDT, go ahead and do it!

2. The technology exists! If you read the "Top Nine Osteoporosis Jaw-Droppers" (page 9) you already know about the tremendous and growing issue of osteoporosis, and all that it forebodes. This issue stretches the current limits

of our resources—including our technologies. We need all osteoporosis instrumentation, and its operators, out there now, in abundance. Do we have enough DXA's in place to cover the need? No. So why not use—and enhance the usage of—one of the most important technologies that we already have at our disposal? How could we not want to broaden our usage of UBDT—on this basis alone?

3. There is no need to wait. I often hear from some who choose not to have a UBDT done: "Well, I'm not yet due for my next DXA. So I will choose to wait until I am due, or wait until my doctor orders it again." Here is an alternative way of viewing this situation: If you do have some possible bone strength loss here, and if the UBDT result happens to show a T-Score that provokes concern in some way, then wouldn't it be wise to spend a small amount of money and time to ensure your good health? Since UBDT is quick and comfortable, why would you wait? Show yourself that your health is important to you!

4. UBDT is safe. Along with DXA, the safety of UBDT is not in question. Not at all.

5. UBDT is quite affordable. Some mobile programs are offering very inexpensive UBDT, to the point that third-party payer issues become non-issues. (Some programs are even offering UBDT for free). As a provider of these tests, I know that they will cost you no more than an average of $15 or $20. This is a small price to pay when it comes to your health.

6. UBDT is accessible. UBDT is convenient, especially if it is taking place at a location that you often frequent. UBDT requires less training and regulation than DXA, thus making it available to address the increasing need for osteoporosis prevention.

7. There is no need for doctors. No clinics, medical centers, hospitals, or white coats are often ever seen with UBDT.

8. We can watch the effects of supplements and behavior changes. In a matter of a few months, we can measure improvements in bone density from taking dietary supplements. We also know several behavior changes that will lower our risk of osteoporosis. This means that if we take the supplements and/or practice the suggested behavior changes, we can use frequent UBDT's to watch our T-scores improve. These improvements show up earlier on UBDT's than on DXA's. (See Chapter 6 for details on my recommended dietary supplement and behavior changes).

9. More frequent monitoring is often recommended. Some leading professionals in the field now feel that the conventionally recommended two-year span between bone density measurements is too long. I strongly agree. Because DXA tests tend to be expensive and inconvenient, the recommended increased frequency can easily be achieved with simple, affordable, and practical monitoring with regular UBDT's. In fact, as a result of a U.S. Food & Drug Administration ruling in 1998, the International Society for Clinical Densitometry now endorses certain UBDT machines for safe and effective bone density monitoring.

10. UBDT offers better counseling and education. Compared to DXA (or avoiding bone density testing altogether), UBDT offers higher quality and more frequent in-depth counseling and education that we need to address this pandemic.

11. Increased testing will promote better outcomes. More people getting more frequent UBDT's will help promote awareness of the prevalence of the disease and turn it

into a commonly discussed public health topic. This will lead to even more optimal diagnostics and care (i.e., DXA's and proper medical care).

12. UBDT acts as a backup for a potentially delayed DXA. Since DXA's are often performed no more often than every two years, they may end up getting delayed or even overlooked at times. For instance, you may experience personal finance changes, changes in insurance, circumstances in your coverage that cause a delay or even reconsideration of a DXA, time constraints, attention to a greater priority at that time, change in doctors for whatever reason, etc. Having regular UBDT's at your convenience makes a lot of sense.

13. The earlier we catch the problem the better. We are seeing loss of bone mass (which can lead to early-onset osteoporosis) in younger and younger people. A 2008 study by the University of Surrey and the Royal Cornwall Hospital in Truro showed a dramatic increase in the number of women in their twenties who have low bone mass (20% of the women tested presented this condition). Many of them would never know to start testing their bone density before the age of 50. By testing younger people with UBDT, we will likely detect many surprise bone density problems—and early detection often allows time to make lifestyle changes in order to prevent further damage. If nothing else, we will have created some awareness and perhaps some useful encouragement or validation, with little expense. Unlike DXA, UBDT has none of the drawbacks you must consider in assessing cost-benefit of over-screening.

ASK DR. KEN:
How Often Do I Need UBDT Done?

Consider this. Let's say that, for whatever reason, your general bone density determination is worsening. Of course you would want to find out about this deterioration as soon as possible after it got started. Certainly the lower your T-Score the more this is a concern.

We know that once a person's bone density starts to decline, that "free fall" can be detectable in as little as six months. But it you are only doing DXA monitoring every two years, you can miss this onset of decline by a long shot. With this possibility out there, it just makes sense to regularly monitor your bone density.

The good news is that you can screen for bone density changes with much more frequency and ease with UBDT! Following are my UBDT[1] recommendations for women over 50 and men over 65 [2]. Please note that they are valid so long as a DXA has not been done within the last six months and a

---

1   Bear in mind, the recommendations I put forth here are for UBDT's. They are not for DXA's. DXA's have their own system of determination.

2   While I do not make specific recommendations for people under these ages, new research is beginning to show that around age 30 people should at least be aware of osteoporosis prevention practices. See Chapter 3 for more on this.

DXA is not already scheduled for sometime in the next three months:

1. If the most recent, valid DXA or UBDT performed on a particular individual showed HIGH fracture risk (i.e., osteoporosis), a UBDT is likely needed no more than **six months** after that last testing.

2. If the most recent, valid DXA or UBDT performed on a particular individual showed a BORDERLINE OR MODERATE fracture risk (i.e., borderline or low bone density, ˙ formerly known as "osteopenia"), a UBDT is likely needed no more than **nine months** after that last testing.

3. If the most recent, valid DXA or UBDT performed on a particular individual showed LOW fracture risk (i.e., normal bone density), a UBDT is likely needed no more than **12 months** after that last testing.

ASK DR. KEN:
Where Can I Get UBDT Done Conveniently?

You can find UBDT in many clinics and major pharmacies, at health fairs and wellness events, at some warehouse grocery stores (e.g., Costco), etc. You should be able to easily locate a UBDT site by going online or making a few phone calls.

The options to explore include:

1. Look for a "Lifeline" location near you: www.lifeline-screening.com, 1-800-449-2350.

2. Find out if your worksite health or insurance company (e.g., "Life Health" at www.lifehealthcorp.com, 303-730-1902) offers bone density screenings through your employer. If not, ask why not.

3. Ask a local chiropractor or two who is doing UBDT in your area.

4. Call G.E. Lunar, Hologic, Norland, or Wallach Surgical for the contact information of their regional representative. Call that individual and identify who in your area uses UBDT.

5. Go to www.nikken.com for some assistance contact-
    ing a Nikken leader in your area who might know who
    is performing Ultrasound Bone Density monitoring of
    "Osteodenx® effectiveness and progress." Some of the
    company's local bone health events have UBDT onsite;
    simply call ahead. If the provider does not plan to have it
    at the next event, ask if he or she could arrange to do so
    if you would agree to attend. And if that does not get you
    to one, ask who in your community is providing UBDT as
    a regular service. (More information about Osteodenx®
    appears in Chapter 6.)

I am confident that as more people become aware of
UBDT effectiveness, the number of options for UBDT will
increase.

ASK DR. KEN:
What Are the Risk Factors for Osteoporosis?

We know of nine basic causes of osteoporosis and its current pandemic:

1. **Hormone imbalance:** When a woman becomes post-menopausal (or peri-menopausal), her blood estrogen level becomes lower. Bone mass begins to decrease along with that.

2. **Inactivity indoors:** Many of us get too little exercise—especially the all-important weight-bearing activity (walking, running, and other "impact" forms of movement) and weight resistance. However, forms of fitness that promote balance (increased muscle tone) are also important because good balance can help you avoid or mitigate serious falls. If you are getting less of these activities than what is considered moderate or reasonable, then you are running the risk of under-exercising. If you are also regularly staying indoors you are probably not getting enough ultraviolet energy to produce the Vitamin D you need in order for your bones to absorb sufficient levels of calcium (see below). This important vitamin is rightfully getting more and more attention from researchers and physi-

cians as to its broadscale significance. Being inactive and staying indoors too much often go hand in hand.

3. **Deficiency of dietary nutrients** (minerals and anti-oxidants): Whether or not you believe, as most do (but not all[1]), that we tend to be deficient in calcium, no one disputes that calcium is among the minerals that our bones need to remain strong. And we can take dietary supplements to increase our calcium intake. In addition, I believe that much more will soon be known about the role of antioxidants and they will be assigned more and more importance toward creating and maintaining bone health and bone strength.

4. **Smoking:** The more you smoke, the more of an osteoporosis risk factor you carry.

5. **Animal protein overload:** This includes meat (of all animals) and dairy. The idea runs counter to popular belief because dairy products are supposed to be good for our bones, right? I believe that the dairy industry may well have contributed to our current osteoporosis problem in many ways. I am not alone in my suspicions here. But that story is for another day.

Do I think everyone should become a vegetarian or vegan? I am not sure (see Chapter 7 for more on this). But I know that moderation—in many areas of life—is often a sensible practice. So over the long haul, make a rule and a habit to try to go easy on the animal protein.

6. **Demographics** (race, gender, family history, fracture history, bone structure, age): Caucasians and Asians are at greater risk for osteoporosis. It also runs in families. Women are at greater risk overall (though men can certainly get osteoporosis as well). Having had a previous

---

1 The 2008 book ***The Calcium Lie*** by Robert Thompson, M.D., certainly disputes whether such a broadscale public calcium deficiency truly does exist.

fracture now places you at greater risk for another. Being small-boned is also a risk factor. Older individuals are more at risk than younger ones.

Perhaps post-menopausal, older, Caucasian and Asian women who are small-framed, who have broken more than a couple bones in their past, and who have osteoporosis in their family history, should be more concerned about their bone health than others. But everyone deserves good health and hope for improvement, and most should have UBDT done now.

7.   **Digestive problems:** Some feel that osteoporosis is often a digestive problem.[2] This warrants attention if such problems are clearly obstructing your ability to absorb and therefore utilize the necessary nutrients you need for proper bone health. Certain digestive conditions (e.g., lactose intolerance, untreated celiac disease, inflammatory bowel disease, and gastro-esophageal reflux disease) may play an important role in what could ultimately result in a high fracture risk. How much of a factor this is in most general cases, however, is not quite clear at this time.

8.   **Toxic substances in our daily lives:** Caffeine, alcohol, sodium, and perhaps unidentified environmental toxins[3] are accepted as established risk factors for osteoporosis. Some specific medications are also problematic, including corticosteroids, thyroid medications, and many others (see Appendix B for more information).

Carrier proteins that are responsible for carrying calcium and other elements to bone can get occupied by carrying toxic elements instead. We have a limited supply of those carrier proteins.

---

2   Johns Hopkins Health Alerts: http://www.johnshopkinshealthalerts.com/reports/back_pain_osteoporosis/3043-1.html

3   The exact identities of these are unknown or unconfirmed at this time.

But many questions remain unanswered: Are these substances normal for us to consume, and considered naturally "tolerable" or "less significant" by the human body as true toxins? How many of these indirectly, and over time, actually cause a dehydrated state; is dehydration really the issue instead? We do know that bone, as a mineral bank for important bodily systems, will accept even toxic (or heavy metal) elements into our boney structure. Does that weaken our bones?

9. **Aging:** This one is even more unclear. Most experts do not consider osteoporosis a normal and natural part of aging. So, do we believe the majority who say that most people need to increase or maintain their calcium intake over time? Or are we to instead believe the minority who say that we are typically getting too much calcium and that it is causing a number of other medical conditions because of its abundance (thus we are more likely to be deficient in other bone-strengthening minerals)?

Well, new research published in the world's premier journal for bone health, Osteoporosis International (January 2009) suggests that both of these arguments may in fact be correct! The research shows that perhaps the issue is instead one of "transport" to the joints, and thus to bone, through carrier proteins once the body absorbs the calcium.

Enriched Lactoferrin (ELF) is a carrier protein that the body makes, and it makes less of it as we get older. The consequence of that creates issues with osteoporosis, kidney stones, sleep problems, inflammation, and perhaps even the #1 killer, heart disease. But recent research has demonstrated success with bone strength blood markers being increased by new, purified forms of natural ELF through over-the-counter oral supplementation.

The proprietary name for ELF as a dietary supplement is Osteodenx°. Nikken, Inc., a research and development company, brought this breakthrough product to market and combines it with calcium supplementation and Vitamin D. Osteodenx® has none of the disadvantages of most pharmaceuticals, is all-natural, and may well be more effective than many of the pharmaceutical options. Further, many who are taking Osteodenx® will state emphatically that it eliminates the need for prescription medicines. I believe that Osteodenx®, or Enriched Lactoferrin supplementation, could well represent the future of optimal osteoporosis supplementation and care.

I personally have screened many people on Osteodenx®, and quite honestly am impressed with the T-scores I have seen. In fact, both my wife and I are on Osteodenx®. If we are addressing aging in the process, and perhaps deterring it, great!

A sign that I usually place in very close proximity to my UBDT machine when screening:

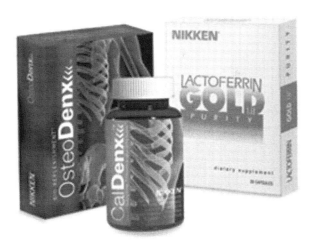

This is called the Osteodenx® BONE HEALTH PACK.

I have been directly testing people who are taking various supplements, and I know that this one **does** work!

FOR STRONGER BONES, THINGS TO AVOID

Remember: The more of these that you can avoid, the better your chances of never getting (and even overcoming) osteoporosis.

- ∾ Smoking
- ∾ Excessive alcohol intake
- ∾ Excessive caffeine intake (coffee, tea, sodas, etc.)
- ∾ Excessive protein intake
- ∾ Excessive sodium intake
- ∾ Sedentary lifestyle
- ∾ Being indoors all (or almost all) of the time
- ∾ Exposure to particular medications (see Appendix B), as well as to certain other environmental toxins
- ∾ Significantly delaying your decision to have at least one bone density test (because for where you are—and where you are going—to be so much more meaningful, you must know where you started)

See Appendix C, the Sundial of Osteoporosis Prevention, for a summary illustration of how to get it right.

ASK DR. KEN:
How Does Being a Vegetarian or Vegan Seem to
Affect Overall Bone Strength?

Please note that I use the terms "vegan" and "vegetarian" interchangeably. Here I am really referring to the strict vegetarian (technically, vegan): those who do not eat eggs, dairy products, or fish. Most people are familiar with the word "vegetarian" but not always "vegan."

As I said in Chapter 6, I do not endorse either a vegetarian or a non-vegetarian diet. Here's why:

First of all, though conflicting, evidence seems to suggest now that vegetarians—overall—seem to enjoy a higher bone mineral density than do non-vegetarians. Thus, vegetarians are at lower risk for osteoporosis and low bone density.

(By the way, you might ask: "If I am expected to have a better-than-average UBDT score, why the extra need to have the test? Well, this is why: You have an opportunity to show your great score to others. Yes, it is something to enjoy, and to be proud of! It also proves that all your efforts and beliefs are indeed working. Your vegetarian lifestyle choice works for you!)

Second of all, many physicians and researchers say that a vegan's calcium intake is as sufficient as a non-vegan's. Some say that it is not. Some say that it simply does not matter.

Some say that a better "quality" of bone from a vegan's diet is more likely to occur than from that of a non-vegan. Some even say that calcium is actually in too great a supply for dietary intake—that most are getting too much, and that minerals, dehydration, and particular aging factors are really what is at work here (see Chapter 6 for more on this). So, I believe that it is fair to conclude that calcium intake may very well be a non-issue in this discussion.

So, the following are the findings that appear, at this point, to be relevant.

Concerning attaining/sustaining bone strength, a vegan's apparent advantages over a non-vegan are:

1. Much lower animal protein intake

2. Possibly a healthier gastro-intestinal tract to facilitate better absorption of calcium and/or other minerals, along with a possibly higher Vitamin D absorption rate

3. Likelihood of better intake of antioxidants (although antioxidants are not yet confirmed to be bone-strengtheners)

Concerning attaining/sustaining bone strength, a vegan's apparent disadvantages over a non-vegan are:

1. In general, a smaller body frame than a non-vegan

2. Overall, a smaller variety of Vitamin D^3-containing food choices (non-vegans can choose fatty fish, eggs, and meat to get their Vitamin D^3)[1]

---

1   The difference between Vitamin D^2 and D^3 is the issue here. Vitamin D^2 comes from yeast, and in some cases from elements derived from ultraviolet-irradiated mushrooms. Vitamin D^3 is synthesized by our skin or is manufactured from lanolin (derived from sheep) or fish oil

   The bulk of current research indicates that the beneficial effects of Vitamin D^3 supplementation could well be absolutely enormous. Bone strength improvement does appear to be one of those many positive and profound benefits. Is Vitamin D^2 good enough for the purpose of gaining optimal bone health? It appears that it may well fall short in being able to perform—for all of us—in the ways that D^3 appears to.

3. Possibly a greater tendency to avoid the more relevant supplements and/or fortified foods for improved bone density (though this fact is somewhat unclear at this point)

"Bones tell stories."
— Unknown

*Five Hurdles for Many or
One Simple Step for Everyone*

In closing, I want to emphasize that five things MUST occur for anyone to have a DXA scan:

1. You must want to have it done.

2. Your doctor must want you to do it as well! It simply will not take place in the absence of the required doctor's order.

3. Your insurance company must also want you to have it.

4. Your budget must allow a DXA scan to take place.

5. Your schedule must allow time to obtain the necessary approvals, get a DXA screening appointment onto your calendar, and then go to the appointment.

With UBDT, there are no "five hurdles". With UBDT, you just.....do it. Get a small amount of money from your pocket. Have a seat. Complete a very short form. Ask any questions. Take your shoe and sock or stocking off. Allow for only a few minutes out of your busy day. Relax. Just....do it.

Because of the five hurdles to being tested for osteoporosis using the DXA approach, it is obvious that all those who need to be tested are not being reached. We are overcomplicating the current major method of osteoporosis testing at a time when the problem seems to be spreading. We need to be simplifying the screenings in as many ways as possible. Clearly, all technologies that are available to us now must be employed. They must be utilized towards the solution. Now.

We know that 7 of 10 people who have osteoporosis are not even aware they have it. That means that those 7 of 10 people are not being tested! As we have seen, statistics indicate that only 3 out of 10 are being tested and could justify closer and more practical monitoring. If we finally would make a strong and sincere effort to reach all those who now need to be tested, DXA's alone simply wouldn't be adequate. And this is one of my major points. We must be realistic.

To emphasize our focus on the "7 of 10", UBDT—clearly—would be highly effective in at least helping to address this very important figure. At the present time, we absolutely must go in this direction!

Currently, UBDT is under-utilized and under-appreciated and this needs to end. It is far too important of a solution to the problem of not reaching those with osteoporosis. We are allowing way too much suffering and missing way too many opportunities to serve a greater number of people.

I invite all to look into UBDT—and its science, its usefulness, and its intended application for the mainstream. In fact, do MORE than that. Have it done!

I hope I have helped the cause. I hope I have stimulated some very important awareness here. I hope I have offered acceptable solutions for those in need.

We need UBDT screenings to be done en mass, and we now need that technology to be found, from a practical standpoint, almost everywhere! UBDT represents what could ultimately be a mass approach and a very sound approach, at that. It is time for UBDT's day in the sun.

Appendices

APPENDIX A: MEDICATIONS THAT MAY CAUSE BONE LOSS

These medications may cause bone loss. If you are taking any of them, be sure to ask your doctor about any bone loss concerns. Please note that this list may not include all medicines that may cause bone loss.

- Aluminum-containing antacids
- Anti-seizure medicines (only some), such as Dilantin® or Phenobarbital®
- Aromatase inhibitors, such as Arimidex®, Aromasin®, and Femara®
- Cancer chemotherapeutic drugs
- Cyclosporine A and FK506 (Tacrolimus)
- Gonadotropin-releasing hormone (GnRH), such as Lupron® and Zoladex®
- Heparin
- Lithium
- Medroxyprogesterone acetate for contraception (Depo-Provera®)
- Methotrexate
- Proton pump inhibitors (PPIs), such as Nexium®,

Prevacid®, and Prilosec®
- ∞ Selective serotonin reuptake inhibitors (SSRIs), such as Lexapro®, Prozac®, and Zoloft®
- ∞ Steroids (glucocorticoids), such as cortisone and prednisone
- ∞ Tamoxifen® (premenopausal use)
- ∞ Thiazolidinediones, such as Actos® and Avandia®
- ∞ Thyroid hormones in excess

(Source: National Osteoporosis Foundation: http://www.nof.org/aboutosteoporosis/detectingosteoporosis/medicineboneloss)

APPENDIX B: SUNDIAL OF OSTEOPOROSIS PREVENTION

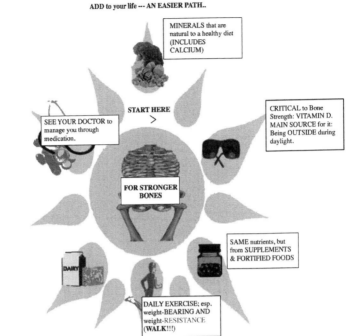

ADD to your life --- AN EASIER PATH..

MINERALS that are natural to a healthy diet (INCLUDES CALCIUM)

START HERE

SEE YOUR DOCTOR to manage you through medication.

CRITICAL to Bone Strength: VITAMIN D. MAIN SOURCE for it: Being OUTSIDE during daylight.

FOR STRONGER BONES

SAME nutrients, but from SUPPLEMENTS & FORTIFIED FOODS

DAIRY

DAILY EXERCISE; esp. weight-BEARING AND weight-RESISTANCE (WALK!!!)

FIVE STAR ON-SITE TESTING; Dr. Kenneth C. Howayeck, Director; 2149 Otis Dr., #333 Alameda, Ca 94501
(925) 858-5696   Dr.Ken@yahoo.com

APPENDIX C: GLOSSARY

Bone density: The amount of bone tissue in a certain volume of bone. Bone Density is often associated with an even more important concept: bone strength. This book uses the terms interchangeably.

Calcium: A mineral found mainly in the hard part of bones, where it is stored. Calcium is essential for healthy bones, and is also important for muscle contraction, heart action, nervous system maintenance, and normal blood clotting. Food sources of calcium include dairy foods, some leafy green vegetables (such as broccoli and collards), canned salmon, clams, oysters, calcium-fortified foods, and tofu.

DXA (an acronym): Dual energy X-ray absorptiometry. It is the most commonly used device to directly assess bone density, which in turn assesses your resistance to fracture.

Hip fracture: Broken bone in the hip, a key health problem among the elderly, usually due to a fall or other trauma involving direct impact to a hip bone weakened by osteoporosis.

Osteoporosis: Thinning of the bones with reduction in bone mass, due to depletion of calcium and bone protein. Osteoporosis predisposes a person to bone fractures.

Stress fracture: A fracture caused by repetitive stress, as may occur in sports, strenuous exercise, or heavy physical labor. Osteoporosis increases the possibility of stress fractures.

T-Score: A comparison of a patient's bone mineral density to that of a healthy thirty-year-old of the same sex and ethnicity. This measurement is used in post-menopausal women and men over age 50 because it best predicts the risk of future fracture.

(Source: Medterms: www.medterms.com)

APPENDIX D: About Five Star Onsite Testing

Five Star Onsite Testing offers screenings by an experienced, personable podiatrist who has no practice or product to promote. We offer screenings upon request at places of employment and a variety of community wellness events.

Features include:

- Use of new, high-quality G.E. Lunar Technology
- Immediate, easy-to-read results reported on the spot
- Three-minute screenings
- Average cost of only $15-$20 per screening

For more information on our services or for scheduling Dr. Howayeck for a speaking engagement, please call: 925-858-5696 or send email to: Dr.KenH@yahoo.com.

Made in the USA
San Bernardino, CA
31 August 2014